Fibromyalgia

The complete guide to fibromyalgia, understanding fibromyalgia, and reducing pain and symptoms of fibromyalgia with simple treatment methods!

Table Of Contents

Introduction 1
Chapter 1: The Growing Burnout Epidemic 2
   What is Fibromyalgia? 3
      Widespread Pain 4
      Incapacitating Fatigue 4
      Impaired Cognitive Functions 4
      Other Symptoms 4
   Fibromyalgia in Women 5
   Causes of Fibromyalgia 5
      Genetics 5
      Infections 6
      Physical Trauma 6
      Fibromyalgia and Pain 6
   What is Chronic Fatigue Syndrome? 7
      Causes of Chronic Fatigue Syndrome 7
      Core Symptoms of Chronic Fatigue Syndrome 8
      What are the Differences between Fibromyalgia and Chronic Fatigue Syndrome? 9
Chapter 2: How to Manage Fibromyalgia Pain 11
   Natural Treatments: 11
   Prescription Relief for Fibromyalgia 13
Chapter 3: How to Cope With Fibromyalgia 17
   Dealing with Sleep Problems 17
   What Can You Do to Relieve Sleep Problems? 17
   Fibromyalgia and Nutrition 19
   Fibromyalgia Exercises 22
Conclusion 25

Introduction

I want to thank you and congratulate you for downloading the book, "Fibromyalgia".

This book contains helpful information about fibromyalgia, what it is, and how you can treat it.

You will learn about how Fibromyalgia is diagnosed, its possible causes, along with treatment methods.

This book explains the signs and symptoms you may experience when inflicted with Fibromyalgia, and provides treatment options for them.

The treatment methods provided include both medical, dietary, and alternative therapies. Ultimately a combination of the different treatment options will result in the best outcome possible.

This book will explain to you tips and techniques that will allow you to successfully understand and limit the discomfort caused by fibromyalgia, and eventually overcome it!

Fibromyalgia can leave you with no energy, and make day to day life difficult. With the help of this guide you will learn to improve and beat the condition, and regain your energy and the lifestyle you deserve!

Thanks again for downloading this book, I hope you enjoy it!

Chapter 1:
The Growing Burnout Epidemic

Do you often feel short of energy, and struggle to make it through the day? Learn how your body creates and spends energy and the reasons why many of us are suffering from the burnout epidemic.

Take a close look at your usual daily routine. Early morning, you munch on cereal or bacon to start your day right, and when mid-morning comes and your energy begins lagging, you may reach for a fast fix such as a cup of brewed coffee, a sugary snack, or even a soda. By mid-afternoon, you may try to replenish lost energy at work by eating energy bars or sipping iced coffee. You may even depend on many types of energy-boosting techniques so that you can push through for the rest of the day.

By following this routine, you may be able to get a lot done. However, once you force yourself to work against fatigue - many times every day for months or even years - you will notice that your health will begin to wane. Eventually, many of the strategies you are relying on to get the energy boost you need could lead you to bad health.

Too much consumption of caffeine and sugar could increase the imbalance of sugar in the blood, causing diabetes and adrenal fatigue. Working for long hours every day and regularly skipping sleep could increase your weight, may cause depression and even affect your mental health. Rather than boosting our body and helping us to become more adept, all these energy-boosting solutions are working against the body's natural mechanisms to attain overall health. They only lead to energy depletion, which sets up our body for even larger energy deficits.

Bear in mind that energy is our capacity to work, to create, to think, to move, and even to enjoy. Energy is what pushes us to exert physical strength and sustain quality of output. Energy also provides mental alertness to solve daily problems. Hence, it is highly recommended that you manage your energy well to achieve a more satisfying life.

It is clear that damaging the body's energy machinery just to gain a short-term boost makes no sense. Unfortunately, many of us do this every day, and we are surprised why life can be very hard to deal with because we feel so exhausted.

Changing your lifestyle to better manage your time and energy can be difficult but doable. All you need is sheer discipline and a lot of hard work to achieve your goals for the day without relying on cheap solutions.

However, all's not fair when it comes to the burnout epidemic. There are cases wherein people feel fatigue, stress, and exhaustion not because of poor energy and time management but because of serious health concerns. Many individuals who feel these symptoms may suffer from fibromyalgia and Chronic Fatigue Syndrome.

What is Fibromyalgia?

Fibromyalgia is a health disorder characterized by muscular and joint pain accompanied by stress, fatigue, and inability to sleep well. Doctors believe that fibromyalgia worsens pain by altering the brain's interpretation of pain receptors.

Take note that fibromyalgia is a syndrome that is characterized by a set of symptoms. Once they are present in one person, they signify the presence of a certain disorder or a disease. With fibromyalgia syndrome, the common symptoms are the following:

Widespread Pain

The pain caused by fibromyalgia is usually characterized by a sustaining dull pain that could last for at least two to three months. Widespread pain means that your body will feel the ache on both sides and above and below your waist.

Incapacitating Fatigue

Individuals who are suffering from fibromyalgia usually wake up feeling exhausted, even though they sleep enough. Sleep can be interrupted by widespread pain, and numerous patients with fibromyalgia also experience sleep disorders including sleep apnea and restless legs syndrome.

Impaired Cognitive Functions

Fibromyalgia is also associated with "fibro fog" that impairs the ability of a person to concentrate, pay attention, and focus on mental tasks.

Other Symptoms

Most patients with fibromyalgia may also experience stress, headache, and cramping in the lower part of the abdomen.

Fibromyalgia in Women

Women are found to be more vulnerable to fibromyalgia. According to the National Institute of Health, about 80% to 90% of patients with this syndrome are women. The reason for this could have something to do with female hormones, genes, and differences in the immune system. However, there is still no established fact why women are at a higher risk of acquiring the disease compared to men.

Causes of Fibromyalgia

Even with numerous advancements in the field of medical research, experts are still clueless about the causes of fibromyalgia. However, doctors believe that the condition may likely involve different factors including genetics, infections, and emotional or physical trauma.

Genetics

Fibromyalgia is not transmitted directly from parents to their children, but the syndrome can appear to cluster within families. The probability of acquiring fibromyalgia is higher in the immediate families of people with fibromyalgia compared to families without the disease.

As a matter of fact, the DNA from family members of patients with fibromyalgia and other chronic pain syndromes have spawned several types of genes that may shed light to the reason why the syndrome can run in families.

These genes play crucial role in the response of the nervous system to pain. Some genes are also linked with anxiety and depression, which could be the reason why specific antidepressant drugs can help in reducing symptoms of fibromyalgia.

Infections

Many patients who have fibromyalgia acquire a viral infection along with it. Patients with active viral infections are at primary risk of getting more infections, specifically bacterial infections that can lead to more severe problems.

Some individuals with fibromyalgia are more susceptible to any kind of infection because the disorder can make them weaker and more at risk of infection. It is crucial for your doctor to determine the different factors to sort out if the infection is the primary cause, an aggravator, or a consequence of the disease.

Physical Trauma

Post-Traumatic fibromyalgia is a specific type of the disorder caused by a physical injury. Doctors who are specializing in fibromyalgia report that most of their patients say that their condition was caused by an injury, about 60% to 70% mostly caused by whiplash injury.

Fibromyalgia and Pain

The pain that is associated with fibromyalgia is widespread, which means you will feel the ache on both sides of the body and above and below the waist. Patients also report certain areas of the body that can feel pain regardless of what drugs you take. Muscles and joints may feel like they have been pulled or overworked although you have not performed any strenuous work. There are instances that the muscles may twitch. Other times, you may feel a burning sensation with deep stabbing pain. Some people with fibromyalgia may experience pain around the joints in their shoulders, neck, hips, and back. This type of pain makes it extra difficult to exercise or sleep.

Fibromyalgia pain is considered chronic because the ache can last much longer than you would normally expect. The pain may seem unending. The enduring headaches, joint pain, neck pain, and back pain can affect healthy sleeping patterns. Inability to sleep well can lead to increased achiness, daytime fatigue, and morning stiffness. Even though you want to do some exercises or be active in the daytime, you may not able to do so because of hip pain, leg pain, knee pain, and other joint aches. These things will incapacitate your ability to work and have fun.

The chronic pain may cause irritation, so the patient may find it difficult to deal with people around them. If the pain is not diagnosed properly, and the person does not seek the right treatment, the symptoms could lead to fatigue, anxiety, irritability, depression, and social isolation.

What is Chronic Fatigue Syndrome?

Chronic Fatigue Syndrome or CFS is considered as the cousin of Fibromyalgia, because the symptoms may appear similar. Similar to fibromyalgia, those with CFS also feel fatigue to the point that they cannot easily complete their usual daily activities. Although CFS has no known cause and can be hard to diagnose, the major symptoms can be cured.

Causes of Chronic Fatigue Syndrome

Even today, doctors are still not certain about the causes of Chronic Fatigue Syndrome. In some cases, CFS manifests after a physical or emotional trauma or after being exposed to toxins. However, there is no known single cause of CFS.

Experts suggest the following are possible causes of CFS: weak immune system, hormonal imbalance, and genes. But it is important to point out that there is no sufficient evidence to establish a solid connection between these causes and CFS.

Core Symptoms of Chronic Fatigue Syndrome

The symptoms for CFS often manifest suddenly. However for some patients, they gradually develop over weeks. The symptoms could change in one day, and there's the tendency that the symptoms will stop abruptly (remission) and then will begin to appear again (relapse).

There's a wide range of symptoms of CFS. However, there is a core set of symptoms that may appear on patients with the syndrome. The following are the core symptoms:

Chronic mental and physical fatigue

The tiredness can be constant or it may stop then start again. The fatigue cannot be relieved by rest, and it can be excruciating to the point that it can affect your daily activities.

Weakness after Being Active

This symptom could mean that you will feel ill or weak after doing strenuous activities such as exercise, running, or swimming. The weakness is not often sudden, and it may take more than a day to regain strength.

Inability to Sleep

The chronic pain could be really severe and cause a person suffering from CFS to not sleep well.

Pain

Pain that is associated with CFS could be widespread or in one place. In some cases, the pain can be isolated in one area then move to another. The patient may experience muscle pain, joint pain, and headaches.

Other Symptoms

A patient with CFS may also experience problems with concentration, short-term memory, sensitivity to light and noise, confusion, and feeling disoriented. In some cases, the patients may also experience dizziness, lightheadedness, shortness of breath when active, nausea, urinating often, irritable bowel syndrome, and weight change.

What are the Differences between Fibromyalgia and Chronic Fatigue Syndrome?

Some doctors treat CFS and fibromyalgia separately, while others may think they are just the same disorder or a variety of the same condition. Research shows that about 65% of people with a diagnosis also fit the criteria for the other.

Fibromyalgia and CFS are known to manifest core symptoms including pain, fatigue, inability to sleep, chronic headache, irritable bowel syndrome, cognitive impairment, dizziness and impaired coordination.

One main difference, when it comes to diagnosis, is which symptom is the worst - fatigue or pain. The diagnosis can be affected by your doctor's familiarity with these diseases, but experts have found key differences. Most cases of CFS show after flu-like symptoms and could be associated to a virus.

CFS patients usually show chronic immune system activation, signifying that the body is fighting the infection, while those with fibromyalgia do not. In addition, the diagnostic criteria for CFS includes sore throat and low-grade fever, while the criteria for fibromyalgia often does not. On the other hand, the onset of fibromyalgia is usually traced to an emotional or physical trauma. The pain associated with fibromyalgia could get better with gentle massage, while the pain for CFS often cannot.

Chapter 2:
How to Manage Fibromyalgia Pain

It's not the end of the world if you are suffering from Fibromyalgia, because pain relief can be achieved. With growing research into the syndrome and better technology, doctors now have a deeper understanding of the condition, and are using different types of medications to treat the core symptoms.

Helping the patient with fibromyalgia to cope with the pain and continue with his or her daily activities is the primary goal of the treatment. The following treatments are often performed to manage the pain associated with fibromyalgia:

Natural Treatments:

5-Hydroxy Tryptophan (5-HTP)

A natural amino acid, 5-HTP helps in creating serotonin, which is a neurotransmitter in the brain that is associated with happiness. Studies reveal that this amino acid can improve symptoms of fibromyalgia such as anxiety, pain, stress, and fatigue. Foods that are rich in 5-HTP are those that are very rich in protein such as fish, beans, meat, and eggs.

Acupuncture

Acupuncture is the ancient Chinese natural healing treatment in which a skilled person will use very thin needles to ease out the pain in specific areas and in the process curing different conditions. A study, co-conducted by the Health Innovations Research Institute, concluded that there is some evidence that the ancient healing art of acupuncture can ease out fibromyalgia pain.

Manual Lymph Drainage Therapy

Manual Lymph Drainage Therapy is a type of massage that helps in moving lymph fluid in the body. The treatment can help the body to eliminate wastes and toxins, but depends on muscle movement to make sure that the system will remain efficient. Rhythmic movements could help in stimulating blood flow and possibly loosening up lymph blockades, which can cause pain.

Meditation

Some rheumatologists believe that meditation can alter the way the brain processes pain receptors, hence improving symptoms. By calming the mind, the body can enter into deep rest and relaxation that may boost the body's natural healing process.

Yoga

Numerous studies show that a regular yoga session could help relieve the symptoms of fibromyalgia. A research conducted by the Oregon Health and Science University revealed that yoga exercises can be effective in reducing pain associated with fibromyalgia.

Bear in mind that the natural remedies described above are alternative treatments for fibromyalgia. It is highly recommended to consult your doctor first before trying anything in your quest to ease out the symptoms of the disorder. Read on to learn more about the prescription treatments to relieve fibromyalgia pain.

Prescription Relief for Fibromyalgia

Relieving the widespread pain of fibromyalgia is the aim of taking medication that your doctor prescribes. However, take note that not every medication works the same way. Some drugs target the central nervous system to suppress pain, while others operate in the muscles to relieve pain.

Aside from treatments that are focused on managing pain, prescription drugs can also work to relieve fatigue, sleep problems and other symptoms such as headaches, bladder discomfort, and irritable bowel. If the patient also suffers from peripheral neuropathy or arthritis, the doctor may prescribe drugs to target particular regional pains.

Take note that the prescription plan should be according to the patient's specific case as well as response to past prescribed treatments. Below is a list of treatment sampling for different symptoms.

Prescription Relief for Pain:

Muscle Relaxation.

Patients with fibromyalgia often have knotted or tight muscles that are difficult to relax. The treatment for the muscle stiffness includes prescription of muscle relaxants such as cyclobenzaprine or tizanidine.

Booster for Brain Chemicals.

Norepinephrine and serotonin work together in the spinal cord and in the brain to ease out pain-related receptors. It is recommended to increase the level of these hormones to enhance the ability of the body to combat pain. Prescription drugs for this treatment include milnacipran and duloxetine. Other similar drugs with higher sedating power include doxepin and amitriptyline, and are recommended to take before bedtime. Even though these drugs are anti-depressants, they are prescribed mainly to ease out pain associated with fibromyalgia.

Opiod Pain Relievers.

Tramodol, the mildest of all opiod analgesics could reduce pain caused by fibromyalgia. Apart from operating as a weak opiod, it also enhances the action of norepinephrine and serotonin to help in reducing discomfort. Dosage can be increased to manage moderate to severe pain.

Dopamine Imitator Medications.

If the body feels pain, the brain releases dopamine to relieve the pain. However, for still uncertain reasons, the dopamine release does not happen when the body is suffering from fibromyalgia. Hence, doctors often benefit from treatment with a dopamine-enhancing drug such as pramepixole.

Slowing Down Pain Signals.

Nerve receptors in the muscles and joints send signals to the brain if there's damage that is often interpreted as pain. Specific anti-epileptic medications such as gabapentin and pregabalin operate to minimize the effects of these signals to alleviate pain caused by fibromyalgia. These medications also help in improving sleep.

Prescription Relief for Fatigue

Chronic fatigue is rated as the second worst symptom after pain. Fatigue associated with fibromyalgia is more severe compared to what people consider as regular weariness, and considerably affects the quality of life. If you feel more fatigue than pain, consult your doctor. There's a possibility that you are low on thyroid hormone, which is often the case with at least 20% of patients and can cause severe fatigue. The good thing is, this condition can be diagnosed through a blood test and the thyroid hormone can be increased through supplements. But if the diagnostic tests turn out to be normal, your doctor may prescribe one of the drugs below to help ease out fatigue.

Alerting Drugs.

Other alerting drugs that work totally different from the serotonin boosters include armodafinil, buproprion, modafinil, and amantadine.

Serotonin Enhancers.

Even though a prescription drug that only enhances serotonin without boosting norepinephrine does not help with the pain, some medications can be highly alerting to ease out fatigue. Examples are escitalopram, fluoxetine, and sertraline.

Prescription Relief for Sleep Problems

Most patients with fibromyalgia wake up in the middle of the night and suffer from an inability to sleep. As a result, their mornings are unrefreshed because they have failed to restore their energy. The following medications are prescribed to fight this symptom:

Insomnia Drugs.

Treatment of fibromyalgia that involves relieving sleep problems usually involves the prescription drugs used for people with insomnia such as eszipoclone, zolpidem, and trazodone.

Restless Legs Syndrome Drugs.

Some patients with fibromyalgia also suffer from restless legs syndrome or also known as limb movements during sleep. Treatment of this symptom may include low doses of pramepixole.

Chapter 3:
How to Cope With Fibromyalgia

Many people with fibromyalgia manage to continue with their daily lives. However, the chronic pain and fatigue linked with the disorder usually make daily activities very difficult. If you are still working, either full-time or part-time, it is crucial to learn about effective management of fibromyalgia symptoms and coping up with its effects on your life.

Dealing with Sleep Problems

Patients with fibromyalgia usually suffer from sleep problems such as insomnia. A more common problem is waking up during the night which interrupts deep sleep. Meanwhile, other sleeping problems such as sleep apnea and restless legs syndrome can also be linked with fibromyalgia.

Many people with fibromyalgia report about awakening in the morning feeling tired with low energy. More often than not, they are more tired in the morning and many go back to bed to relieve their fatigue. In addition, it can be very difficult for fibromyalgia patients to focus during the day. This condition is known as fibro fog.

What Can You Do to Relieve Sleep Problems?

Practicing better sleep practices can help you manage the sleep-related symptoms of fibromyalgia. Enhancing your sleep may help relieve the pain, fatigue, as well as fibro fog. You can try the following sleep enhancing strategies. You can also ask your doctor about prescription drugs that are safe and effective in improving your sleep patterns, as discussed in Chapter 2.

- **Get enough sleep.** Not too much and not too little. Sleep only as you need to be energized for the next day. Eight hours of sleep seems to solidify your energy source while excessive sleep may even lead to fragmented sleep patterns.

- **Keep a sleep journal.** Take note of your sleeping habits every night as well as the triggers that have interfered with your sleep. Review the journal regularly over several weeks so that you can get more insight about your sleep problems.

- **Exercise regularly in the morning and not before bed time.** Research reveals that regular exercise has beneficial effects in achieving a high-quality sleep.

- **Stay away from excessive naps in the morning.** Too many naps can affect your sleeping pattern at night.

- **Set aside a regular time to wake up every day.** A schedule for awakening can help in fortifying the circadian cycling and could lead to improving insomnia.

- **Try relaxation treatments.** Deep breathing, gentle massage, and other relaxation strategies are believed to relieve pain and fatigue.

- **Keep the temperature in your room low**. A warm room cannot put you into deep sleep.

- **Stay away from alcohol or caffeine**, as they both interfere with good sleep.

Fibromyalgia and Nutrition

About 42% of patients with fibromyalgia reported symptoms after eating specific foods, and although much of the research is in the initial stages, there is evidence that simple dietary changes could help patients manage the symptoms, especially pain and fatigue.

Dealing with fibromyalgia can be very challenging, and improvements are usually incremental. Most traditional doctors prefer prescribing medications such as analgesics and antidepressants that may result in side effects.

A physician who is nutritionally oriented is more likely to prefer a more biochemical perspective for a patient with fibromyalgia to determine the underlying problems, which can be treated with safe nutritional therapies. It is true that fibromyalgia is a complex disease with no easy cure. However, when you look at a whole body approach with diet, natural supplements and lifestyle, you can harness the natural healing abilities of your body.

Below are nutritional tips for fibro patients. Just make certain to consult your doctor before you change your diet.

Increase Intake of Vitamin D

Most of us don't get enough Vitamin D, which is essential for patients with fibromyalgia. Deficiency in Vitamin D can be similar to the fibromyalgia symptoms. As such, patients must be screened for deficiency. Research shows that a lack of Vitamin D may cause pain in the muscles and joints, and increasing your intake of Vitamin D could help. Doctors recommend loading up on Vitamin D supplements, particularly during winter. Foods that are rich in Vitamin D are fish oils, mushrooms, whole grain cereals, tofu, and dairy products.

Stay Away from Additives

Food additives such as aspartame and monosodium glutamate (MSG), may act as excitotoxin molecules, which is a chemical group that has the capacity to activate neurons that can increase reception to pain. Experts believe that minimizing intake of additives could help in reducing the symptoms of fibromyalgia.

Load Up on Fish

Fatty fish such as salmon, herring, sardines, and mackerel are rich in Omega-3 fatty acids, which are known to relieve inflammation and can help in preventing cardiovascular diseases. Increasing intake of these certain fishes can help in reducing the pain caused by fibromyalgia. Other foods that are rich in omega-3 fatty acids are walnuts, cereal, oatmeal, and flax seed.

Avoid Caffeine

Because fibro patients usually experience sleep problems, it can be enticing to load up on coffee to get more energy for the day. However, this is not an ideal solution. Some people drink coffee so they can compensate for not getting enough sleep at night. Caffeine can actually cause sleep problems at night. If you drink coffee, especially in the few hours before bedtime, it may interfere with your sleep patterns. Instead of coffee, you can take green tea that is very rich in antioxidants.

Love Veggies

Some doctors believe that oxidative stress causes the symptoms of fibromyalgia. Oxidative stress happens when the body does not generate enough antioxidants to fight free radicals in the body. Fruits and vegetables are rich in crucial antioxidants such as Vitamins A, C, and E that fight free radicals to keep the body normalized.

Get Enough Glutathione

Glutathione is the main antioxidant produced by the body to protect it from oxidative damage and to support the detoxification process of the liver. Studies reveal that fibro patients with low levels of glutathione are more prone to morning stiffness. There are available glutathione pills, but if you want an all-natural diet, you can increase intake of foods such as eggs, cruciferous veggies, and garlic. These foods are very rich in sulfur, which is the primary component of glutathione.

Proteins and Non-Starchy Vegetables

Choosing a diet that is rich in high-quality proteins as well as enough consumption of non-starchy vegetables is a crucial step in reducing the symptoms of fibromyalgia. Vegetables that are non-starchy virtually include all veggies except potatoes. Meanwhile, it is also crucial to reduce intake or totally stay away from foods that are rich in refined sugars and starches such as bread, crackers, cookies, pasta, etc. Foods that are heavy on refined sugar and starches could lead to health problems such as early signs of diabetes, fatigue, and even hypertension.

Fibromyalgia Exercises

It can really be challenging to live with chronic pain, fatigue, and stiffness caused by fibromyalgia. Even though therapy and medication are crucial in managing these symptoms, adding physical activity could greatly improve the quality of your life.

The first thing you need to do is to keep moving. The more you move, the less pain and fatigue you will feel. In addition, exercise can help you to get better sleep and reduce the need to take medications for pain. Below are recommended exercises. Just make sure that you consult your doctor first before starting any program.

Walking

Walking is a great form of mild aerobic exercise that offers several health benefits. It provides oxygen to the muscles to retain their health and function, it helps in boosting stamina and energy, and minimizes pain and stiffness. As a matter of fact, a comprehensive research revealed that mild aerobics is very effective in managing fibromyalgia symptoms. A good alternative to walking is biking. The rhythmic motion helps in relaxing the muscles. Other mild aerobic exercises include water aerobics such as swimming and working on a treadmill.

It is recommended to perform short bursts of walking and not long stretches. Studies show that breaking down a longer workout into short sessions can provide the same health advantages. Doctors generally recommend performing aerobic exercises at least 3 to 4 times a week every other day. You can motivate yourself by encouraging friends to join you in walking or performing aerobics exercises.

Strength Workout

Fibromyalgia patients can do strength training using light weights. The trick is to lift precisely and slowly to enhance the tone of the muscles and to make them stronger. Studies reveal that resistance workouts can help in combating depression. Fibro patients are recommended to work out the chest, legs, back, abs, shoulders, and arms, at least two to three times a week. Begin with a weight that you can lift easily for about eight reps, and then slowly increase the pace to 10 to 12 reps as your progress. Once you can lift the weight a dozen times, and two sessions in a row, you can up the weight, but go back to 8 reps.

In weight training for fibromyalgia patients, it is recommended to shorten the range of motion. In the case of bicep curl, you need to perform two parts. First, you need to bring your hand up to your shoulder, and then you need to lower it back down. The second phase can be the issue as you may feel a bit of discomfort and make pain worse for fibro patients. Curtailing this phase could help in minimizing muscle soreness.

Stretching

Stretching at least once a day can increase your flexibility, enhance range of motion, and loosen up stiff muscles. Eventually, this exercise can help in easing daily movements. Don't forget to stretch during workouts to help you improve your condition. Bear in mind that stretching is done to cool down your body and not for warm up. Hence, you must do stretching exercises after the workout. There's the possibility of hurting your muscles before a workout.

Hatha Yoga

The Hatha Yoga is a type of yoga that combines gentle postures, meditation, and breathing. Experts believe that this can reduce the physical as well as the emotional symptoms of fibromyalgia, especially for women. Regular practitioners of Hatha Yoga reported a considerable reduction of pain and have learned to cope better with the disorder.

Doing yoga can also help the patient to build energy and endurance as well as improve sleep and focus. Aside from Hatha Yoga, you can also practice Tai Chi, in which you need to perform graceful movements. Tai Chi is believed to be a better cool-down workout than stretching.

You can modify the movements to reduce the stress. For instance, if a certain yoga position hurts, you need to modify it to still reap the benefits with less pain. For starters, it is crucial to find a professional instructor who is also familiar with fibromyalgia. You can ask your doctor or physical therapist for good recommendations.

Conclusion

Thank you again for downloading this book!

I hope this book was able to help you learn more about fibromyalgia and its treatment methods!

Bear in mind that acquiring fibromyalgia is not the end of your world. You can still work, have fun, and live your life as long as you know how to manage and cope with fibromyalgia.

The next step is to put this information to use, and begin improving your fibromyalgia condition.

Finally, if you enjoyed this book, please take the time to share your thoughts and post a review on Amazon. It'd be greatly appreciated!

Thank you and good luck!

www.ingramcontent.com/pod-product-compliance
Lightning Source LLC
LaVergne TN
LVHW021750060526
838200LV00052B/3559